For Models & Entrepreneurs
Simply Meal Planning

Aries Ford

BS, RDN, LDN

Register Dietitian Nutritionist

Table of contents

Aries Ford, RDN, LDN is a dietitian, motivational speaker specializing in nutrition conferences and workshops. Aries has over 15 years of experience as a dietitian in planning, implementing and coordinating clinical patient nutritional care to promote health and control various diseases. Aries experience includes but not limited to: Nutrition Support Dietitian, extensive knowledge in counseling individuals and providing appropriate interventions of various disease conditions in clinical, community and nursing home environments. Experience also extends in developing curriculum, teaching groups and evaluating training techniques. A graduate of the University of North Carolina at Greensboro and a Buffalo NY native. Aries also enjoys traveling, being a mother to two handsome boys and appearing on various TV and radio shows in her free time.

SPECIAL THANKS

To Joe Yancey, Founder of MoStyle Magazine and owner of Joe Yancey Studios.

Introduction

Thank you for choosing "Simply Meal Planning". We believe in improving health and wellness for all ages through effective meal planning and activities. Registered Dietitians are the Nutrition experts that change lives. Our focus is to assist you in obtaining your personal wellness goals. We are committed to providing you with the best tools and nutritional foundation to jump start your personal" healthy" lifestyle change, which will boost your over all physical and mental capabilities. We value the individuals we serve and will continue to strive to provide each client with expert quality care.

Chapter 1

This is Why Simply Meal Planning Works

Best results occur with at least 14 sessions over a 6 month period of time according to researchers at Johns Hopkins. Studies also suggest major results are likely when individuals combine and complete the following:

1. Use of scientific diet strategies or use of diet mechanisms that have been proven scientifically through evidence as well as professional guidance.
2. Exercise at least 150 minute moderately weekly. Be sure to consult a physician before newly starting an exercise program.
3. Using behavior strategies and modifications such as tracking food intake and exercise, weekly weights and meal planning.

Chapter 2

You make the pledge to:

1. Follow health care recommendations
2. Keep your appointments to the best of your ability via phone or email
3. Provide honest answers to promote your lifestyle change

I'll make the pledge to:

1. Provide you with accurate evidenced based answers.
2. Treat you with respect.
3. Will not share personal information with other individuals.

Additional suggestions include scheduling medical appointments per your doctor's recommendations as well as keeping track of important health results such as the following:

Height_____, weight_____, waist (inches around)_____,

blood pressure_____/_____

total cholesterol_____,

LDL cholesterol_____,

HDL cholesterol_____,
Triglycerides_____,

blood
Glucose_____,

A1C (if you have diabetes)_____

Chapter 3

Let's discuss your lifestyle change vision and goals. Now let's try our best to succeed!

Your short term goals: _____weight or other_____

Your long term goals:_____weight or other

_____

Chapter 4

Simply Meal Planning

<u>Morning Meal</u>   Time:

_____serving of carbohydrates

_____oz of meat or ___servings of meat
substitutes

_____servings of fat

Snack-time:_____   servings
size_____

 _____grams of Carbohydrates

_____Water

<u>Noon Meal</u>   Time:

_____serving of carbohydrates

_____oz of meat or ___servings of meat
substitutes

_____servings of vegetables

_____servings of fat

Snack-time:_____   servings
size_____

 _____grams of Carbohydrates

_____water

<u>Evening Meal</u>   Time:

_____serving of carbohydrates

_____oz of meat or ___servings of meat substitutes

_____servings of vegetables

_____servings of fat

Snack-time:_____   servings size_____

_____grams of Carbohydrates

_____water

*note-snacks are usually consumed if there is at least a 5 hour time lapse between meals for adults. The dietitian or certified professional will individualize snack serving sizes and choices for children and teenagers with this meal plan for optimal growth and development.

Estimating Portion Sizes

A computer mouse equals about ½ cup

A fist equals about 1 cup

A palm equals about 3 ounces of protein

A thumb equals about 1 ounce

Carbohydrate Example List

1 serving is equivalent to 15 grams of carbohydrate

½ cup cooked cereal

1 slice of bread or bun

½ of a small bagel

6" tortilla

½ cup of corn, beans , potatoes or peas

1/3 cup of rice or pasta

1 cup of soup

3 cups of popcorn

1/3 cup of frozen yogurt

1 small fresh fruit

½ banana

1 cup of fresh berries or melon

¼ cup of dried fruit

½ cup of milk or plain yogurt

Protein and meat substitute Example List

1 serving is of the following

1 oz of lean meat such as chicken, turkey, fish, seafood, beef, pork and lamb

¼ cup of cottage cheese or tuna

2 Tbsp of peanut butter

Vegetable Example List

1 serving is ½ cup cooked or 1 cup raw

Asparagus, green beans, broccoli, cabbage, cauliflower, carrots, celery, cucumber, eggplant, onions, greens, mushrooms, peppers, radishes, spinach, squash, zucchini, tomatoes

Fat Example List

1 serving is of the following

1 tsp of butter, oil, mayo(regular)

1 Tbsp of cream cheese, half and half heavy cream or salad dressing

Recommended fluids: water preferred with meals and snacks. Water can be replaced with one calorie free beverage on occasion. Suggest carbonated water as a substitution for soda and juice.

My Estimated Fluid Intake:

_____8 oz glasses of water daily

Greater results may be achieved by limiting:

1. high fat dairy products such as butter, cream cheeses and regular milk
2. All artificial sweeteners and sugar
3. Breads ,rolls and pasta
4. Fried foods
5. Alcohol
6. Processed foods with artificial flavorings, chemicals, food additives, preservatives

Chapter 5

My Food and Activity Tracker

Date: Time:

State Food or beverage:

Serving size:

Date: Time:

State Food or beverage:

Serving size:

Date: Time:

State Food or beverage:

Serving size:

Date: Time:

State Food or beverage:

Serving size:

Date: Time:

State Food or beverage:

Serving size:

Date: Time:

State Food or beverage:

Serving size:

Date: Time:

State Food or beverage:

Serving size:

Date: Time:

State Food or beverage:

Serving size:

Date: Time:

State Food or beverage:

Serving size:

Date: Time:

State Food or beverage:

Serving size:

Date: Time:

State Food or beverage:

Serving size:

Date: Time:

State Food or beverage:

Serving size:

Date: Time:

State Food or beverage:

Serving size:

Date: Time:

State Food or beverage:

Serving size:

Date: Time:

State Food or beverage:

Serving size:

Date: Time:

State Food or beverage:

Serving size:

Date: Time:

State Food or beverage:

Serving size:

Date: Time:

State Food or beverage:

Serving size:

Date: Time:

State Food or beverage:

Serving size:

Date: Time:

State Food or beverage:

Serving size:

Date: Time:

State Food or beverage:

Serving size:

Date: Time:

State Food or beverage:

Serving size:

Date: Time:

State Food or beverage:

Serving size:

Date: Time:

State Food or beverage:

Serving size:

Date: Time:

State Food or beverage:

Serving size:

Date: Time:

State Food or beverage:

Serving size:

Date: Time:

State Food or beverage:

Serving size:

Date: Time:

State Food or beverage:

Serving size:

Date: Time:

State Food or beverage:

Serving size:

Date: Time:

State Food or beverage:

Serving size:

Date: Time:

State Food or beverage:

Serving size:

Date: Time:

State Food or beverage:

Serving size:

Date: Time:

State Food or beverage:

Serving size:

Date: Time:

State Food or beverage:

Serving size:

Date: Time:

State Food or beverage:

Serving size:

Date: Time:

State Food or beverage:

Serving size:

Date: Time:

State Food or beverage:

Serving size:

Date: Time:

State Food or beverage:

Serving size:

Date: Time:

State Food or beverage:

Serving size:

Date: Time:

State Food or beverage:

Serving size:

Date: Time:

State Food or beverage:

Serving size:

Date: Time:

State Food or beverage:

Serving size:

Date: Time:

State Food or beverage:

Serving size:

Activity Tracker

Day of the week:

Number of minutes:

Type of activity:

Day of the week:

Number of minutes:

Type of activity:

Day of the week:

Number of minutes:

Type of activity:

Day of the week:

Number of minutes:

Type of activity:

Day of the week:

Number of minutes:

Type of activity:

Day of the week:

Number of minutes:

Type of activity:

Day of the week:

Number of minutes:

Type of activity:

Day of the week:

Number of minutes:

Type of activity:

Day of the week:

Number of minutes:

Type of activity:

Day of the week:

Number of minutes:

Type of activity:

Day of the week:

Number of minutes:

Type of activity:

Day of the week:

Number of minutes:

Type of activity:

Day of the week:

Number of minutes:

Type of activity:

Day of the week:

Number of minutes:

Type of activity:

Day of the week:

Number of minutes:

Type of activity:

Day of the week:

Number of minutes:

Type of activity:

Chapter 6

Quick Facts on Food Labels

Don't forget that it is also important to know what's in your food. Let me show you what to look for on a label. Items high in fat will most likely be high in calories. Eating too much fat makes us fat. Healthy eating means reducing the fat and sodium we consume.

Serving size- determines the amount of calories and nutrients in one serving. You have to add more calories if you decide to eat more or the entire package. The same idea goes for fat, sodium and carbohydrates as well.

Fat grams- Compare products and choose foods with the least amount of total fat grams- less than 5 grams of fat per serving for snack foods.

Sodium- Try to choose foods lowest in sodium. 140mg is a good goal per serving.

Carbohydrates- One serving of carbohydrates is equivalent to 15 grams of carbohydrates. A sugar gram is just a component of carbohydrates. Carbohydrates break down into sugar.

Fiber- Try to choose items with 5 grams or more per serving.

NOTES:

Chapter 7

Success Advantage and Focus Setting

Consultation Session # -1 2 3 4 5 6 7 8 9 10 11 12 13 14 15 (circle the session at the end of contact)

Next appt date and time_____

 Next appt date and time_____

Next appt date and time_____

 Next appt date and time_____

Next appt date and time_____

Next appt date and time_____

Next appt date and time_____

 Next appt date and time_____

Next appt date and time_____

Next appt date and time_____

Next appt date and time_____

Next appt date and time_____

Next appt date and time_____

Next appt date and time_____

Next appt date and time_____

Next appt date and time_____

NOTES:

DISCLAIMER

This book is designed as a tool to promote optimal health as well as individualized meal planning in collaboration with a dietitian or other certified professional. Please consult your primary care physician before starting an exercise or diet plan.

Recommended Readings and References

Selections from the Academy of Nutrition and Dietetics, research studies at Johns Hopkins and the CDC

Other beneficial publications that will enhance your knowledge and help you reach your goals include:

- Healthier, Happier and Well!
- Happier Kids! Raising Children to Eat Better and Be More Active.
- 14 Days Your Way

VISIT **ARIESFORD.ORG**
for more information and a
complete listing of other
publications

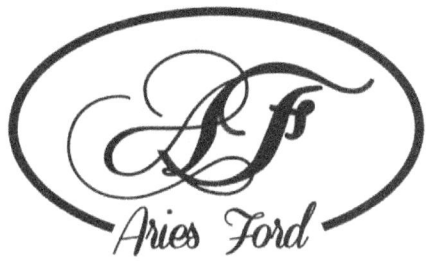